The Complete
Keto Diet Cookbook
for Beginners #2019

Lose Weight with Fast and Easy Keto Diet Recipes
incl. 4 Weeks Weight Loss Plan

[1st Edition]

Jerry Chandler

Table of Contents

EXCLUSIVE BONUS!

Get Keto Audiobook for FREE NOW!*

*The Ultimate Keto Diet Guide 2019-2020:
How to Loose weight with Quick and Easy Steps*

SCAN ME

or go to

www.free-keto.co.uk

Introduction

What is the keto diet?

"Keto" is short for "ketogenic" which represents focusing on larger portions of fat instead of carbohydrates. The usual weight loss diets we follow actually take away the fats and replace them with a higher ratio of carbs. Keto diet does the exact opposite and encourage taking fatty dishes. That is why you will feel much happier on a keto diet and will have less cravings for snacking.

Advantages of a keto diet

Weight Loss

Typically, a weight loss program will force you to stay away from all the yummy fatty dishes. Not this diet! A ketogenic diet inspires you to find pleasure in the food you eat and benefit from it at the same time.

Due to our ordinary food habits, our body uses carbohydrates as the main source of energy. The keto diet changes that priority and encourages our body to utilize fats for energy instead. This way more fats are burned up which reduces our overall weight significantly.

Ketogenic diets result in much more productive results compared to other diet forms. The weight, as well as the BMI (Body Mass Index), waist-hip ratio and body fat percentage go down much more effectively. This diet is also a lot more sustainable. You can hold onto it for a long time compared to low-fat diets.

Blood Sugar Control

Keto is an incredibly helpful diet for diabetic patients and those individuals who show similar tendencies. It has the power to lower your blood sugar levels naturally through the correct food selection. Compared to low-fat diets, this has proved to be more effective in bringing the sugar levels down.

This diet keeps the carbohydrate intake under control. Carbs are responsible for high blood sugar. When we eat food items rich in carbohydrate, our body breaks it down into sugar which then enters the blood. As a result, the more carb we eat, the more sugar gets into our bloodstream. This, in turn, encourages the pancreas to store a lot of the blood sugar for energy.

By switching to the keto diet, we limit these carbs and force our body to break down fats instead. It maintains a healthy level of glucose and prevents spikes in blood sugar. Using different sweeteners instead of sugar in keto dishes also helps the purpose.

Enhanced Focus

Concentrate better with the ketogenic lifestyle. This diet enhances your mental focus every single day by preventing blood sugar spikes. Such a controlled approach keeps the brain sharp enabling it to focus better.

The fatty acids form a major part of the keto diet. These acids are used by our brain as an alternative energy source to carry out its complex functions faster. This particular energy source named ketone can feed up to 75% of your brain's energy.

Because of this gigantic effect of fatty acids on our brain, the keto diet helps sharpen our mind in the long run. As a result, it has the ability to prevent and reduce the intensity of neurogenic diseases such as Parkinson's and Alzheimer's.

Higher Energy

After the initial struggle, keto diet has proved to be very helpful in maintaining an energetic lifestyle. As we mentioned before, it is more sustainable than other diet alternatives. Compared to carbs, fats are much more effective as physical fuel. The fat molecules enhance your energy levels during the day.

Epilepsy Cure

The origins of the keto diet rest in an effort to find an epilepsy cure. Almost a century ago, the keto diet was suggested to epileptic patients which brought successful results.

Epilepsy is the result of abnormal brain activities. It causes your nervous system to experience sudden irregularities. As a result, the patient undergoes unpredictable seizures frequently. It can also cause muscle spasms, unconsciousness and convulsions. To battle epilepsy, Dr. Russel Wilder came up with this carefully crafted keto diet in 1924.

A 1998 study proved the effectiveness of keto diet in epileptic children. 34% of the subjects experienced 90% fewer seizures after three months of switching to the keto diet. In recent years, such studies have been performed on adult patients. They have shown similar results proving the success of keto diet yet again.

Blood Pressure Improvement

Keto diet is more equipped to optimize blood pressure compared to other diets. Blood pressure is basically the force moving blood exerts on the blood vessel walls.

The American Heart Association suggests an ideal blood pressure for humans should be 120/80 mm Hg. If the numerator (systolic BP) ranges from 120-139 mm Hg and the denominator (diastolic BP) ranges from 80-90 mm Hg, that person has prehypertension. If someone's blood pressure continues to be higher than 140/90 mm Hg, that person can be in grave danger.

A 2007 study conducted on 300 individuals over a year revealed how keto diet can decrease both their systolic and diastolic blood pressure effectively. Thus, adopting a ketogenic lifestyle can improve your blood pressure levels and help you reach its optimum state.

Cholesterol Improvement

Cholesterol is often demonized by the majority. However, it actually has both good and bad editions. There are two types of cholesterol called LDL and HDL. Your body needs to balance these two so that the LDL cannot enter your bloodstream. The small particle LDL can cause heart issues by building up along the artery lining.

Keto diet can increase the ratio of pattern A LDL or the "good" cholesterol. As a result, it makes the LDL less likely to be oxidized and create the artery build-up. This diet also reduces triglycerides which is responsible for strokes.

Reduce Hunger and Cravings

Ketosis has a significant impact on your metabolism. It keeps breaking down fat molecules instead of carbohydrates in order to get the required energy. As a result of this process, ketone bodies are formed which effectively suppress the appetite. Ketone bodies are well-known for controlling satiating hormones and making you feel full on a daily basis. Because of this, you hardly feel snacking and restrict your daily food intake to a healthy amount.

Free from Acne

This diet can improve your skin conditions noticeably. Studies have shown in the past how skin inflammation reduces once you switch to a keto diet. In consequence, the people suffering from acne can get rid of those protrusions and marks naturally.

You can enhance the skin even further by reducing dairy food items in your daily diet. There are different clinical and home-made procedures available to keep your skin clean as well.

Battles Cancer Growth

Recently, researchers have been turning to keto diet for battling cancer growth. For example, some London-based scientists started discovering the effectiveness of keto diet as an alternative therapy for malignant brain cancer. It increases plasma ketone bodies and reduces plasma glucose levels. This functions strongly against the growth and density of tumours.

What am I allowed to eat and what is prohibited?

Before you go out for buying the groceries, take a look below. Go through our lists of food items showing which are good for your keto diet regime and which are not.

YES to these:

Low-carb Vegetables

Like all good diets, the keto diet also needs a strong base of vegetables. Veggies are the staple for maintaining a healthy body and metabolism. Since this diet is based on low carbohydrates, low-carb vegetables are its staple.

Vegetables, in general, are a great source of all the important nutrients for your body. Every meal of the day should incorporate them. The vegetables which are low on carbohydrates tend to be very rich in vitamins, minerals, fibre and antioxidants. They can build a sturdy skeleton to add huge amounts of fat later on for a ketogenic diet.

We recommend low-carb vegetables like spinach, cauliflower, bell peppers, cabbage, brussels sprouts, eggplant and arugula. However, remember to avoid starchy options like potatoes, carrots, beets and turnips.

Low-sugar Fruits

Fruits are generally a no-no for keto diets since they naturally possess so much of sugar. However, there are some fruits which contain only a little bit of sugary elements. Thus they can make a great addition to your keto groceries and add more flavour to the regular dishes.

The one thing you must be careful about is the quantity. Although they are low on sugar, you still need to restrict their intake on a daily basis. The stars of such fruits are raspberries, avocados and olives. Besides, blackberries, coconut, lemon and tomatoes are also quite valuable for keto diet routines.

Seafood

Although most of the sea creatures are still a mystery, the ones we have discovered so far are great additions to a keto diet. Seafood tends to be much higher in proteins compared to livestock options. They also contain a great amount of omega-3 fatty acids - one of the best source of healthy fats.

Shrimp, salmon and tuna are at the heart of many delicious heavy dishes. They also make quite the companion for healthy salads at office lunch. Along with these three, you can include crab, cod, mackerel, mussels and sardines for an occasional burst of seafood flavour.

Meat

Another good source of protein is meat. There is a wide spectrum of meat products we can find at our local grocery stores now. Each of them has its own share of nutritional advantages. Not to mention, they taste delicious and add lovely flavours to an otherwise bland dish.

Since meat is high in both fat and proteins - the two main targets of a keto diet - we rely on them a lot. The most common meat variations we find include beef, chicken, turkey, pork and lamb. Remember to only invest in organic poultry and grass-fed beef. They ensure the high quality of fat composition which in turn adds to your healthy regime.

Eggs

No one can deny eggs since it can be prepared in numerous ways. No matter how you cook it, eggs taste delicious in all forms. They are also very helpful for ketogenic diet regime since every egg has roughly 6g protein and 1g carbohydrate. That ratio makes eggs ideal for keto diet.

Moreover, they help to activate beneficial hormones which keep your appetite in control all day long. You will not feel the sudden cravings for desserts or snacks regularly. If you have spiking blood sugar levels, eggs can also make them stable again. With all these factors working together, your overall calorie intake will reduce every day.

Remember to eat the whole egg, not just whites. Most of its nutrients are embedded in the yolk. You will miss out on powerful antioxidants if you cut the yolk out every time. Antioxidants like lutein and zeaxanthin help to protect the vision. On the contrary, the LDL cholesterol keeps your heart safe from diseases.

Nuts

Nuts have very high fat and very low carbohydrates by nature. That makes nuts an ideal component for keto dishes. Like the egg, nuts can keep heart diseases away. Additionally, it keeps you away from other chronic diseases like depression and cancer.

Almonds and walnuts are among the most nutritious nut variations available. Besides, Brazil nuts, Macadamia nuts, walnuts, pistachios and hazelnuts are also good choices. If you are feeling hungry, you can just have 5-6 of these nuts and feel full till the next meal.

Seeds

Seeds have high fiber and protein. They have very low portions of carbohydrates in them. That is why seeds are often used to prepare keto dishes. Popular options for seeds include chia seeds, flaxseeds, sesame seeds and pumpkin seeds. Especially flaxseeds have zero gram net carbs. The other three also have a trivial amount of carbohydrates (1-4 gram net carbs).

Dairy

With dairy products, you can have multiple vital nutrients at the same time. They are packed with protein, calcium and healthy fats. They also come in many varieties allowing you to explore your culinary skills. Popular healthy dairy products include cheese, yoghurt, butter and cream.

Oils

Oils are essential to cook most of the dishes. They also carry importance in a keto diet routine since they are rich in healthy fats. Among the wide range of oils available right now, we recommend coconut oil, olive oil (preferably extra-virgin), MCT oil and avocado oil. Keep a few of them just to add new flavours to your keto dishes every day!

Condiments

Condiments enhance the flavour of each dish or add a new twist of their own. The problem with investing in condiments is that most of them are highly processed. So while purchasing them, make sure to check out the nutritional values and look for "no added sugar". The condiments which can help in a ketogenic diet are mustard, ketchup, olive oil mayonnaise and oil-based dressings.

Snacks

The keto diet helps to suppress appetite in a healthy way. However, if you still feel the need to snack in between meals, we have some safe suggestions for you. Go for low-carb crackers, sugar-free jerky, nut butter and dried seaweed.

You can take these anywhere for a quick snack - be it office or study tour.

Caffeine

Everyone needs a shot of caffeine in order to prevent drowsiness. If you are having problems with low energy, you can always rely on tea and coffee. Just be sure they aren't sweetened. A warm cup of tea or coffee in the morning will boost you up for the day. We also shared some caffeine recipes below to help you explore new tastes.

Chocolate

Who doesn't love chocolate? It is hard to resist nibbling on a delicious chocolate bar every now and then. You can have them while on the keto diet too. However, there is one restriction - you can only have dark chocolate. If you still want to try other chocolates, make sure they are 70% cocoa at a minimum.

NO to these:

Sugar-rich foods

This is a no brainer. While you are on keto diet which focuses on healthy fats, you cannot ruin the balance by investing in sugary foods. So you must bid adieu to soft drinks, fruit juices, candies, cake and ice-cream. Oh, don't get disheartened! We got you covered with our dessert recipes below.

Grains and Starches

Food items which primarily depend on wheat or corn like rice, cereal and pasta are a complete no-no. This list of harmful foods also includes most flours except the ones made out of nuts. That is why a keto diet includes many dishes using shredded cauliflower as rice.

Sugary Fruits

Except for the fruits we mentioned in the above section, almost all other fruits are forbidden for keto diet. That is because they are naturally too rich in sugar and can hamper your healthy progress.

Beans

Kidney beans, lentils, peas, chickpeas and all sorts of ingredients falling into this category should be left out of keto diet.

Root Vegetables

Root vegetables contain high amounts of starch and carbohydrates. As a result, they cannot be part of keto diet routines. You need to avoid potatoes, carrots, sweet potatoes and parsnips.

Low-fat Items

This diet is based on food rich in fat. So low-fat items are definitely on the "avoidable" section. They are very high in carbohydrates and are also highly processed.

Alcohol

Alcohol includes a considerable amount of carbs. That is why consuming alcoholic beverages can get you off track. So stay away from them while you are on the diet.

How do I prepare for my keto diet?

Practice Cooking

To be on the keto diet, you will need to let go of the processed foods. Consequently, you will need to set some time aside to cook the items yourself. So practice cooking for a week or two before investing in the keto diet.

Know about Potential Side Effects

Keto diet can cause some side-effects like the keto flu. This is the time period when your body is transitioning from its usual carb-burning routine to the new fat-burning one. It will take 7-10 days for this effect to go away. Within this time you may feel extremely fatigued.

Increase Electrolytes

During the process of ketosis, your kidney gets rid of the water and electrolytes more than usual. As a result, the overall electrolyte level of your body may decrease. So remember to take food rich in sodium and potassium to balance it out. Eat salty foods and non-starchy veggies for a start.

RECIPES

BREAKFAST

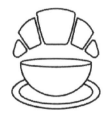

English Muffins

Serves 6| Time: 15 minutes

Net carbs: 40% (1g / 0.03oz), Fiber: 12% (3g / 0.1oz) | Fat: 62% (15g / 0.5oz), Protein: 21% (5g / 0.18oz) | Kcal: 160

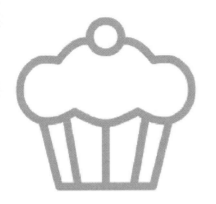

Ingredients:

♦ 4 eggs

♦ 2 pinches of salt

♦ 1 teaspoon baking powder

♦ 6 tablespoons of butter

♦ 4 tablespoons coconut flour

Preparation:

1. Mix baking powder, salt and coconut flour in a bowl.

2. Whisk the eggs into this mixture. Let is sit for a while.

3. Turn the heat to medium-high and melt the butter. Fry six portions of this mixture separated in two batches there.

4. Flip the pieces after two minutes.

5. En muffins with butter.

Biscuits and Gravy

Time: 35 minutes | Serves 8

Kcal: 360, Net carbs: 6% (3g / 0.1oz) | Fiber: 0% (0g / 0 oz) , Fat: 67% (33g / 1.16oz) | Protein: 27% (13g / 0.46oz)

Ingredients:

- 10 ounces crumbled pork sausage
- 1 cup chicken broth
- 1 cup of almond flour
- 1 cup of coconut cream
- 2 tablespoons of cold coconut oil
- 1 teaspoon of coconut oil spray
- 4 egg whites
- 1 teaspoon of garlic powder
- Salt
- Pepper

Preparation:

1. Whisk the egg whites well to achieve the fluffy texture.
2. Mix baking powder and almond flour in another bowl.
3. Cut up the cold butter. Add this and the salt into the flour-powder mixture.
4. Carefully pour the mixture into the egg whites.
5. Place several portions of this dough on the greased cookie sheet.
6. Bake the biscuit doughs for about 15 minutes.
7. To prepare the gravy, cook sausage at medium heat. Stir the cream cheese and broth slowly. Cook it under boiling point for 2 minutes. Add pepper and salt for seasoning.
8. Top each half of a biscuit with ⅓ cup gravy while serving.

Goat Cheese Omelet with Vegetables

Time: 25 minutes | Serves 1

Kcal: 340, Net carbs: 4% (2g / 0.07oz) | Fiber: 2% (1g / 0.03oz), Fat: 56% (28g / 1oz) | Protein: 38% (19g / 0.7oz)

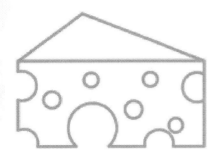

Ingredients:

♦ 1 ounce goat cheese
♦ ½ ounces baby spinach
♦ ¼ sliced scallion
♦ 1 tablespoons of whipped cream
♦ 2 chopped green asparagus
♦ 2 large eggs
♦ ½ tablespoons of butter
♦ Salt
♦ Pepper

Preparation:

1. Whisk the cream and eggs in a bowl together.

2. Fry the asparagus briefly in a nonstick pan with butter. Then move it in another bowl retaining the melted butter.

3. Turn the heat down and add the egg mixture. Once its centre is set, add pepper and salt according to taste.

4. Place the cooked asparagus and spinach on half of this omelette. Sprinkle the goat cheese on it.

5. Flip its other half and cook for about two minutes.

French Pancakes

Time:15 minutes | Serves 2

Kcal: 690, Net carbs: 4% (4g / 0.14oz) | Fiber: 3% (3g / 0.1oz), Fat: 75% (68g / 2.4oz) | Protein: 17% (15g / 0.5oz)

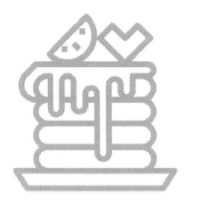

Ingredients:

♦ 4 eggs
♦ 1 ½ ounces of butter
♦ 1 tablespoons of psyllium husk powder
♦ Quarter cup of water
♦ 1 cup of heavy whipped cream
♦ ⅛ teaspoons of salt

Preparation:

1. Combine the eggs, cream, salt and water in a bowl.

2. Add in the husk powder to make a consistent batter. Let it marinate for ten minutes.

3. Pour in ½ cup of batter to make one pancake at medium-high heat.

Upma

Time: 25 minutes | Serves 4

Kcal: 250, Net carbs: 20% (8g / 0.3oz) | Fiber: 10% (4g / 0.14oz), Fat: 52% (21g / 0.74oz) | Protein: 18% (7g / 0.3oz)

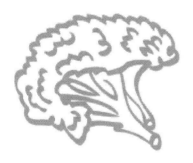

Ingredients:

♦ 15 ounces cauliflower florets, pulsed

♦ 3½ ounces chopped onions

♦ 1½ ounces salted peanuts

♦ ⅓ ounces ginger

♦ 2 tablespoons of mustard seeds

♦ 4 tablespoons of butter

♦ 2 tablespoons of cumin seeds

♦ 2 green chilli peppers

♦ 10 curry leaves

♦ Cilantro

Preparation:

1. Cook the seeds of cumin and mustard in butter. When they begin to sizzle, add in the onions, ginger, curry leaves, peanuts, pepper and salt.

2. Now add the cauliflower pieces and fry the concoction.

3. Add some water to cover the mixture. Cover, stir and cook for approximately 10 minutes.

4. When the water has completely evaporated, serve with some fresh cilantro.

Pumpkin Spice Latte

Time: 5 minutes | Serves 1

Kcal: 215, Net carbs: 4% (1g / 0.03oz) | Fiber: 4% (1g / 0.03oz), Fat: 88% (23g / 0.8oz) | Protein: 4% (1g / 0.03oz)

Ingredients:

- 2 teaspoons of instant coffee
- 1 teaspoon of pumpkin pie spice
- 1 cup boiling water
- 1 ounce unsalted butter

Preparation:

1. Blend everything for 30 seconds. When you see a foam forming, pour in a cup and serve fresh!

Scrambled Eggs with Veggies and Coconut Oil

Time: 5 minutes | Serves 4

Kcal: 250, Net carbs: 20% (11g / 0.4oz) | Fiber: 5% (3g / 0.1oz), Fat: 44% (24g / 0.85oz) | Protein: 30% (16g / 0.6z)

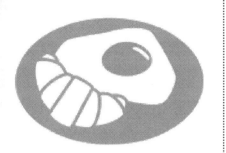

Ingredients:

- 2 tablespoons of frozen vegetables
- 3 eggs
- ½ cup spinach
- Salt and pepper
- 2 tablespoons of coconut oil

Preparation:

1. Heat up the coconut oil and fry the vegetables in it for a while.
2. Add the whisked eggs, spices and spinach to the concoction.

Cornbread

Time: 30 minutes | Serves 4

Kcal: 238, Net carbs: 3% (1g / 0.03oz) | Fiber: 14% (5g / 0.18oz), Fat: 64% (23g / 0.8oz) | Protein: 20% (7g / 0.3oz)

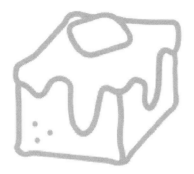

Ingredients:

♦ 2 eggs
♦ 1½ ounces of melted butter
♦ ¾ teaspoons of baking powder
♦ 2 tablespoons water
♦ 2 tablespoons of coconut flour
♦ ⅛ teaspoons of salt
♦   cup whey protein isolate
♦   cup coconut oil
♦   cup oat fibre

Preparation:

1. Take a bowl and mix the dry ingredients in it.

2. Then add the butter, coconut oil, water and eggs into the mixture. Beat it up and add corn extract at last.

3. Bake this mixture for20 minutes in a hot greased cast iron skillet.

Overnight Coconut Chia Pudding

Time: 15 minutes | Serves 1

Kcal: 200, Net carbs: 43% (17g / 0.6oz) | Fiber: 8% (3g / 0.1oz), Fat: 38% (15g / 0.5oz) | Protein: 13% (5g / 0.18oz)

Ingredients:

- ¼ cup of chia seeds
- 1 cup of full-fat coconut milk
- ½ tablespoon of honey
- Fruits and nuts toppings

Preparation:

1. Combine honey, chia seeds and milk in a bowl or jar. Refrigerate it overnight.
2. If the chia seeds appear to be gelled, your pudding is done. Top it with any fruits and nuts you prefer before serving.

Chai Latte

Time: 5 minutes | Serves 6

Kcal: 130, Net carbs: 6% (1g / 0.03oz) | Fiber: 0% (0g / 0 oz), Fat: 88% (14g / 0.5oz) | Protein: 6% (1g / 0.03oz)

Ingredients:

♦ 3 tablespoons of chai or tea

♦ 6 cups of water

♦ 1 cup heavy whipped cream

Preparation:

1. Boil the water and brew the tea in it. Pour it into a cup before the taste turns bitter.

2. Warm the cream up in an oven. Add it to the tea while serving.

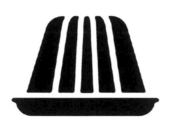

LUNCH

Bacon and Olive Quiche

Time: 45 minutes | Serves 6

Kcal: 410, Net carbs: 10% (6g / 0.2oz) | Fiber: 3% (2g / 0.07oz), Fat: 58% (34g / 1.2oz) | Protein: 28% (16g / 0.6oz)

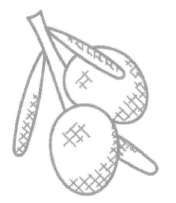

Ingredients:

- ◆ 12 eggs
- ◆ 15 diced olives
- ◆ 6 diced bacon slices
- ◆ ¾ cups of coconut cream
- ◆ 4 cups spinach (chopped)
- ◆ ¼ cups of chopped basil leaves
- ◆ 2 tomatoes (diced)
- ◆ 1 onion (diced)
- ◆ 2 bell peppers (diced)
- ◆ 3 tablespoons of coconut oil
- ◆ 3 garlic cloves (minced)
- ◆ Salt
- ◆ Pepper

Preparation:

1. Sauté the bacon in coconut oil. Move it into a bowl.
2. Sauté onion and bell pepper dices in the bacon fat. Then add the spinach and cook for a couple of minutes.
3. Combine the eggs, olives, tomatoes, basil, bacon, garlic, coconut cream, spinach mixture, salt and pepper. Bake it for 30 minutes.

Salmon and Avocado Salad

Time: 10 minutes | Serves 2

Kcal: 575, Net carbs: 5% (4g / 0.14oz) | Fiber: 8% (7g / 0.3oz), Fat: 58% (49g / 1.76oz) | Protein: 29% (25g / 0.9oz)

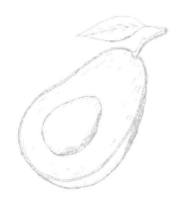

Ingredients:

- 8 ounces of salmon fillet (cooked and flaked)
- 2 tablespoons of lemon juice
- 3 ounces of arugula leaves
- 1 teaspoon of Dijon mustard
- ¼ cup of olive oil (extra virgin)
- 1 avocado (diced)
- Black pepper

Preparation:

1. Combine salmon, arugula and avocado in a bowl.
2. To prepare the dressing, mix vinegar, lemon juice, olive oil, Dijon mustard and black pepper.
3. Toss the salad with a little bit of this dressing and serve fresh!

Cauliflower Potato Salad

Time: 40 minutes | Serves 12

Kcal: 300, Net carbs: 13% (5g / 0.18oz) | Fiber: 5% (2g / 0.07oz), Fat: 70% (27g / 0.95oz) | Protein: 13% (5g / 0.18oz)

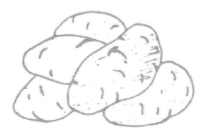

Ingredients:

- 6 large eggs (hard-boiled)
- 8 cups diced cauliflower florets
- 1cup diced white onion
- 1½ cup avocado mayonnaise
- 1 cup diced Dill pickles
- ½ cup diced celery
- ¼ cup mustard (yellow)
- 2 tablespoons of olive oil
- ¼ teaspoon of black pepper
- 1 tablespoons of apple cider vinegar
- ½ teaspoon of sea salt
- Paprika

Preparation:

1. Coat the diced cauliflower with olive oil, pepper and salt. Put them on a baking sheet in one layer and bake for 30 minutes.
2. Dice four of the hard-boiled eggs.
3. Mix everything but the eggs. Now use it to toss the cauliflower and diced eggs. Add salt and pepper for taste.
4. Transfer the salad onto the serving dish. Slice the other two eggs as you please to use them as toppings.
5. Chill and serve with paprika.

Turkey with Cream Cheese Sauce

Time: 25 minutes | Serves 4

Kcal: 790, Net carbs: 6% (7g / 0.3oz) | Fiber: 0% (0g / 0 oz), Fat: 57% (67g / 2.36oz) | Protein: 37% (43g / 1.5oz)

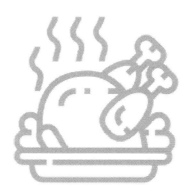

Ingredients:

- ♦ 2 cups of heavy whipped cream
- ♦ 20 ounces of turkey breast
- ♦ 7 ounces of cream cheese
- ♦ 2 tablespoons of butter
- ♦ ⅓ cup of small capers
- ♦ Pepper and salt
- ♦ 1 tablespoon of tamari soy sauce

Preparation:

1. Marinate the turkey with pepper and salt.
2. Warm 1 tablespoon of butter in an oven-proof pan and fry till it becomes golden brown. Put it in the oven and bake until the temperature becomes 74°C.
3. Take remaining liquid of pan into a saucepan. Now stir in heavy cream and cream cheese to it. When it reaches the boiling point, turn the temperature down and let it simmer. You can use tamari sauce to add more flavour.
4. Sauté the capers in remaining butter until they turn crispy.
5. Serve the cooked turkey with sauce and fried capers.

Fish Cakes with Avocado Lemon Dip

Time: 15 minutes | Serves 6

Kcal: 70, Net carbs: 9% (1g / 0.03oz) | Fiber: 18% (2g / 0.07oz), Fat: 63% (7g / 0.3oz) | Protein: 9% (1g / 0.03oz)

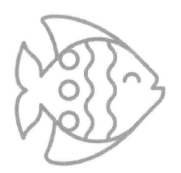

Ingredients:

♦ 1 lb white boneless fish
♦ 2 ripe avocados
♦ ¼ cup of cilantro
♦ 2 garlic cloves
♦ 2 tablespoons of coconut oil
♦ 2 tablespoons of water
♦ Juice of one lemon
♦ Salt
♦ Chilli flakes

Preparation:

1. Blend the fish, garlic, chilli, salt and herbs with a blender. Make 6 patties out of it.

2. Coat a large pan with coconut oil at medium-high heat.

3. Cook the patties until both sides of each piece have turned golden brown.

4. Blend the avocados, lemon juice, water and some salt to prepare the creamy dip.

5. Serve the fish cakes with lemon avocado dip.

Tuna Salad with Poached Eggs

Time: 20 minutes | Serves: 2

Kcal: 760, Net carbs: 5% (6g / 0.2oz) | Fiber: 3% (3g / 0.1oz), Fat: 66% (70g / 2.5oz) | Protein: 28% (30g / 1.1oz)

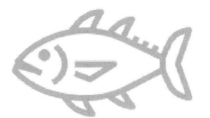

Ingredients:

- 4 ounces of drained tuna
- 4 eggs
- 2 ounces of lettuce
- 2 ounces of cherry tomatoes
- ½ lemon (juice and zest)
- ½ of red onion
- ⅓ cup chopped celery
- ½ cup mayonnaise
- 2 tablespoons of olive oil
- 2 tablespoons of small capers
- 2 teaspoons of white vinegar
- 1 teaspoon Dijon mustard
- Salt
- Pepper

Preparation:

1. Combine the tuna with celery, onion, mayonnaise, mustard, lemon juice, caers, olive oil, salt and pepper.

2. Add vinegar and salt to slightly boiling water. Crack the eggs one by one into the swirling water. Simmer it for two minutes. Take the eggs out with a spoon.

3. Add lettuce and tomatoes to the tuna mix. Serve this salad with the poached eggs and a drizzle of olive oil.

Cabbage Soup

Time: 50 minutes | Serves: 10

Kcal: 260, Net carbs: 10% (4g / 0.14oz) | Fiber: 5% (2g / 0.07oz), Fat: 44% (18g / 0.6oz) | Protein: 41% (17g / 0.6oz)

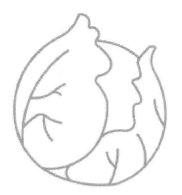

Ingredients:

♦ 10 ounces of tomatoes (diced) and green chilis

♦ 2 lbs. of 90% lean ground beef

♦ 1 chopped cabbage

♦ ¼ diced onion

♦ 4 cups water

♦ 4 cubes bouillon

♦ 1 teaspoon ground cumin

♦ Salt

♦ Pepper

Preparation:

1. Cook the ground beef till it turns brown on medium heat.

2. Add the diced onions and cook till it turns translucent. Move the mixture to a stockpot.

3. Add diced tomatoes, green chilis, bouillon cubes, cabbage, garlic, cumin, garlic and water to it. Mix well.

4. Turn the heat down and cook for 45 minutes.

Indian Chicken Lettuce Wraps

Time: 20 minutes | Serves 2

Kcal: 550, Net carbs: 4% (5g / 0.18oz) | Fiber: 2% (2g / 0.07oz), Fat: 32% (36g / 1.27oz) | Protein: 48% (50g / 1.76oz)

Ingredients:

- 8 lettuce leaves
- 1 lb. of boneless skinless chicken thighs
- 1 cup of cauliflower rice
- 2 garlic cloves (minced)
- ¼ cup of minced onion
- ¼ cup plain coconut milk yoghurt
- 3 tablespoons of ghee
- 2 teaspoons of curry powder
- 1½ teaspoons salt
- 1 teaspoon of black pepper

Preparation:

1. Cut up the chicken into one-inch pieces.
2. Heat up 2 tablespoons of ghee in a pan and cook onions in it until they turn brown.
3. Add chicken, garlic and salt to this concoction. Stir frequently for about seven minutes.
4. Now add the remaining ghee, cauliflower rice and curry powder.
5. Place this delicious chicken curry mix into each lettuce leaf and serve!

Cheesy Taco Skillet

Time: 20 minutes | Serves 6

Kcal: 270, Net carbs: 20% (9g / 0.3oz) | Fiber: 5% (2g / 0.07oz) | Fat: 16% (7g / 0.3oz) | Protein: 60% (26g / 0.9oz)

Ingredients:

♦ 3 cups spinach

♦ 1 lb. lean ground beef

♦ 12 ounces diced tomatoes with green chilis

♦ 2 diced bell peppers

♦ 1 diced yellow onion

♦ 1½ cup shredded cheddar cheese

♦ 2 diced zucchinis

♦ 2 tablespoons of taco seasoning

Preparation:

1. Cook the beef till it turns light brown and scramble it. Burn the excess fat.

2. Now add the vegetables to this beef and cook until they turn brown.

3. Add tomatoes, taco seasoning and the greens. You can also add water for better coating. Combine all these well.

4. Spread the cheese and let it melt.

5. Serve with rice, lettuce or taco - the choice is yours!

Drumsticks with Chili Aioli

Time: 50 minutes | Serves 4

Kcal: 700, Net carbs: 2% (2g / 0.07 oz) | Fiber: 1% (1g / 0.03 oz), Fat: 50% (56g / 2oz) | Protein: 38% (42g / 1.48oz)

Ingredients:

♦ ⅔ cup mayonnaise

♦ 2 lbs. chicken drumsticks

♦ 1 garlic clove (minced)

♦ 1 tablespoon of tomato paste

♦ 2 tablespoons of coconut oil

♦ 1 tablespoon of Tabasco

♦ 2 tablespoons of white wine vinegar

♦ 1 tablespoons of smoked chili powder

♦ 1 teaspoon of salt

♦ 1 teaspoon of paprika powder

♦ Olive oil

Preparation:

1. Place the drumsticks in a plastic bag to marinate.

2. Combine coconut oil, tomato paste, Tabasco, vinegar, paprika powder and salt. Put the mixture into the bag and shake for about ten minutes.

3. Smear the baking dish with olive oil and bake the marinated drumsticks for half an hour.

4. Mix garlic, chilli and mayonnaise to prepare the chilli aioli.

5. Serve the drumsticks with chilli aioli.

DINNER

Caprese Chicken

Time: 40 minutes | Serves 4

Kcal: 313, Net carbs: 3% (2g / 0.07 oz) | Fiber: 2% (1g / 0.03 oz), Fat: 33% (19g / 0.7oz) | Protein: 62% (36g / 1.27oz)

Ingredients:

- 5 chicken thighs (Boneless)
- 2 tablespoons of avocado oil
- 6 ounces sliced mozzarella
- 1 sliced tomato
- ¼ cups of chopped basil
- Salt and pepper

Preparation:

1. Marinate the chicken with pepper and salt. Cook them in simmering oil until each side turns golden brown.

2. Place them in one layer on a glass baking pan. Put tomato slices and mozzarella over the chicken.

3. Bake for 26 minutes. Let the broiler brown the top portion of cheese within two minutes.

4. Serve the delicious caprese chicken with basil.

Shrimp and Sausage Skillet

Time: 5 minutes | Serves 4

Kcal: 330, Net carbs: 8% (5g / 0.18oz) | Fiber: 3% (2g / 0.07 oz), Fat: 37% (23g / 0.8oz) | Protein: 52% (32g / 1.13oz)

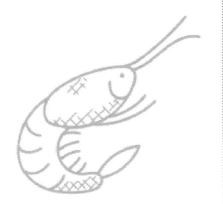

Ingredients:

- ½ lb. sliced green beans
- 12 ounces sliced chicken sausage
- 1 lb. of deveined shrimp
- ¼ cup avocado oil
- 1 sliced red pepper
- 1 garlic clove (minced)
- 1 teaspoon Cajun seasoning
- Salt and pepper

Preparation:

1. Fry the shrimp in 2 tablespoons of simmering avocado oil for a couple of minutes.

2. Add the seasoning over it and cook for a couple of minutes.

3. Sauté the sausage in the remaining oil for about three minutes. Add garlic and jalapeno to it. Now sauté for 30 seconds more.

4. Add the pepper and green beans now. Cook till everything becomes tender.

5. Add salt and pepper for seasoning. Then put back the cooked shrimp and serve warm.

Spaghetti Squash Casserole

Time: 1 hour 25 minutes | Serves 6

Kcal: 430, Net carbs: 8% (5g / 0.18 oz) | Fiber: 3% (2g / 0.07 oz), Fat: 44% (29g / 1 oz) | Protein: 45% (30g / 1.1 oz)

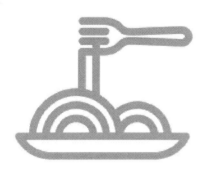

Ingredients:

♦ 1 lb. ground beef
♦ 1 halved and deseeded spaghetti squash
♦ 6 ounces cheddar (shredded)
♦ 2 teaspoons Worcestershire sauce
♦ 4 chopped bacon slices
♦ 2 tablespoons of sugar-free ketchup
♦ 2 minced garlic cloves
♦ ½ teaspoon salt
♦ ½ teaspoons pepper

Preparation:

1. Bake the squash in an oven preheated to 400-degrees Fahrenheit for 40 minutes.

2. Cook the bacon on a pan in medium flame till it turns crisp. Then move it in a bowl.

3. In the same skillet, cook the beef for 6 minutes and crumble it with a spoon.

4. Now add the garlic, pepper and salt. Cook it for 2 more minutes.

5. Take the flesh out of the squash. Now stir in the ketchup, sauce and squash into the beef concoction.

6. Spread cheese on top and put the cover on. Cook for about five minutes on low heat.

7. Serve it with crispy bacon on top.

Mongolian Beef

Time: 6 hours 10 minutes | Serves 4

Kcal: 415, Net carbs: 2% (1g / 0.03 oz) | Fiber: 2% (1g / 0.03 oz), Fat: 40% (25g / 0.9oz) | Protein: 57% (36g / 1.27oz)

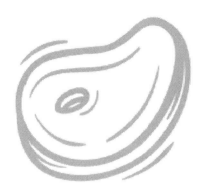

Ingredients:

- 1½ lbs. sirloin steak, sliced
- 2 garlic cloves (minced)
- ⅓ cup of Swerve Brown
- 2 green onions (chopped)
- 2 tablespoons of sesame oil
- ¼ cup tamari sauce
- ¼ cup water
- ½ tablespoon of ground ginger
- ¼ teaspoon red pepper flakes
- ½ teaspoon of glucomannan powder
- Sesame seeds

Preparation:

1. Take a slow cooker and place the sliced beef at its bottom.
2. Mix Swerve Brown, tamari, water, sesame oil, red pepper flakes, garlic and ginger in a bowl. Add the mixture with beef and cook for 5 hours at low temperature.
3. When the beef is cooked, take out a little bit of its broth and place in a bowl. Combine it with the glucomannan powder and return this mixture into the pot.
4. Spread the chopped onions and sesame seeds on top before serving.

Garlic Butter Salmon

Time: 27minutes | Serves 4

Kcal: 450, Net carbs: 6% (4g / 0.14oz) | Fiber: 3% (2g / 0.07 oz), Fat: 36% (24g / 0.85oz) | Protein: 55% (37g / 1.27oz)

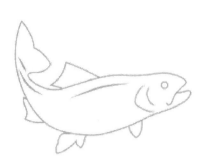

Ingredients:

- 1 lb. cauliflower florets
- ¼ cup of butter
- 1½ lbs. quartered salmon fillet
- 2 tablespoons of chopped parsley
- 1 teaspoon of grated lemon zest
- 3 garlic cloves (minced)
- Salt
- Pepper

Preparation:

1. Melt 2 tablespoons of the butter on a rimmed baking sheet in a preheating oven.

2. Now put the florets of cauliflowers on it. Use pepper and salt to season them. Bake for about ten mintues.

3. Mix garlic with the rest of the butter, lemon zest and parsley to prepare the garlic butter.

4. Marinate the salmon fillets with garlic butter, pepper and salt. Bake until you can flake the fillets with a fork without much effort.

Chicken Quesadillas

Time: **35 minutes | Serves 4**

Kcal: 403, Net carbs: 8% (5g / 0.18 oz) | Fiber: 5% (3g / 0.1 oz), Fat: 41% (26g / 0.9 oz) | Protein: 46% (29g / 1 oz)

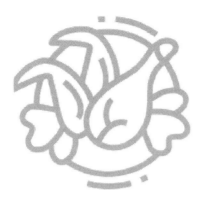

Ingredients:

- 2 chopped boneless chicken thighs
- 48-inch pizza crusts
- 2 green onions (sliced)
- ½ chopped green pepper
- 1 tablespoons of taco seasoning
- 1½ cups cheddar cheese (shredded)
- 2 tablespoons of avocado oil

Preparation:

1. Sauté the chicken in 1 tablespoons of avocado oil for 5 minutes.

2. Spread some taco seasoning on top. Now add the onions and pepper. Cook for five minutes. Transfer it to a bowl.

3. Heat up ½ tablespoons of avocado oil in a pan and place one pizza crust in it. Top it with ½ cup of cheese and half of the cooked chicken mixture in two separate layers. Now put another layer of ¼ cup cheese and one more pizza crust over it.

4. Put the cover on and cook for about 3 mintues. Cook for 2 more minutes after you flip it.

5. Cut it in pieces and enjoy. Repeat the process with other ingredients as well.

Greek Shrimp

Time: 35 minutes | Serves 6

Kcal: 174, Net carbs: 11% (4g / 0.14 oz) | Fiber: 3% (1g / 0.03 oz), Fat: 29% (10g / 0.35 oz) | Protein: 57% (20g / 0.7 oz)

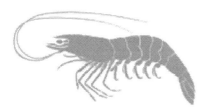

Ingredients:

- 15 ounces of diced tomatoes
- 1½ lbs. deveined shrimp
- ½ cup of grated parmesan cheese
- 2tablespoons of avocado oil
- ¾ cup of crumbled feta cheese
- 2 minced garlic cloves
- ½ teaspoon red pepper flakes
- 1 teaspoon of salt
- ¾ teaspoons black pepper

Preparation:

1. Quick fry the garlic in avocado oil for half a minute in an oven-proof pan.
2. Add tomatoes, salt, pepper flakes and pepper. Cook for 5 minutes.
3. Place the shrimp in one layer on top of this mixture. Sprinkle half of the feta cheese and all of the parmesan cheese on top. Bake it for 13 minutes.
4. Serve the freshly baked shrimp with rest of the feta cheese.

Bacon Brie Frittata

Time: 25 minutes | Serves 1

Kcal: 325, Net carbs: 4% (1.8g / 0.06 oz) | Fiber: 0.2% (0.08g / 0.01 oz), Fat: 58% (26g / 0.9 oz) | Protein: 37% (17g / 0.6 oz)

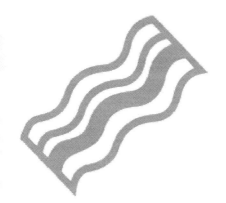

Ingredients:

- 8 eggs (large)
- 4 ounces sliced brie
- 8 chopped bacon slices
- 2 minced garlic cloves
- ½ teaspoon of pepper
- ½ cup of whipped cream
- ½ teaspoon of salt

Preparation:

1. Quick fry the bacon till it turns crisp. Drain it and keep 2 tablespoons of of this bacon grease. Use this liquid to coat the interior of a skillet.

2. Combine ⅔ of the crispy bacon with eggs, cream, salt, pepper and garlic. Cook this in the coated skillet for 10 minutes straight.

3. When the frittata is done, top it with brie slices and rest of bacon. Broil it for 5 minutes at a high temperature.

Asian Steak

Time: 40 minutes | Serves 6

Kcal: 279, Net carbs: 4% (2g / 0.07 oz) | Fiber: 2% (1g / 0.03 oz), Fat: 40% (17g / 0.6 oz) | Protein: 53% (23g / 0.8 oz)

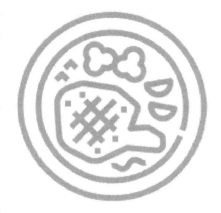

Ingredients:

- 1½ lbs. sirloin steak, diced
- 2 minced garlic cloves
- ¼ cupsoy sauce
- 2 tablespoons of sesame oil
- 2 teaspoons toasted sesame seeds
- 1 tablespoons of sweetener
- ¼ teaspoons red pepper flakes
- cilantro
- ½ teaspoons ground ginger

Preparation:

1. Mix sweetener, soy sauce, red pepper flakes, ginger and garlic in a bowl. Use this mixture to marinate the steak bites for half an hour.

2. Heat up 1 tablespoons of sesame oil on a skillet. Spread the steak mixture in one layer on it. Cook it for about two minutes on each side. Take it out and repeat the process with rest of the steak.

3. If there is any remaining marinade, cook it for 5 minutes and use it as dressing.

4. Serve the steak bites with cilantro and toasted sesame seeds.

Loaded Cauliflower

Time: 20 minutes | Serves 6

Kcal: 200, Net carbs: 10% (3g / 0.1 oz) | Fiber: 7% (2g / 0.07 oz), Fat: 57% (17g / 0.6 oz) | Protein: 27% (8g / 0.3 oz)

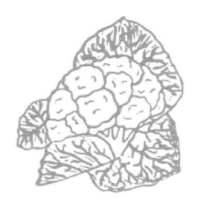

Ingredients:

- ♦ 1 lb. cauliflower florets
- ♦ 3 tablespoons of butter
- ♦ 4 ounces sour cream
- ♦ 1 cup grated cheddar cheese
- ♦ 2 crumbled slices cooked bacon
- ♦ 2 tablespoons of snipped chives
- ♦ ¼ teaspoons garlic powder
- ♦ Salt
- ♦ Pepper

Preparation:

1. Take an oven-safe bowl and put the florets in it. Pour 2 tablespoons of water here and microwave till they become tender. Then drain and let it sit for a couple of minutes.

2. Break down the cauliflower using a food processor.

3. Add butter, sour cream and garlic powder to bring out a creamy texture all over.

4. Transfer this mashed cauliflower to a bowl. Add chives, half of pepper, salt and cheddar cheese to it. Combine all the elements well.

5. Use the remaining cheese and bacon as toppings for the loaded cauliflower. Microwave again to melt the cheese and quickly serve it.

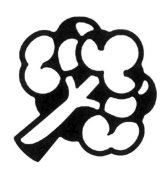

SNACKS & DESSERTS

Chocolate Muffins

Time: 40 minutes | Serves 8

Kcal: 110, Net carbs: 18% (3g / 0.1 oz) | Fiber: 6% (1g / 0.03 oz), Fat: 60% (10g / 0.35 oz) | Protein: 18% (3g / 0.1 oz)

Ingredients:

- 9 tablespoons of melted cocoa butter
- 4 tablespoons of sweetener
- 2 teaspoons apple cider vinegar
- 3 eggs (pastured)
- 1 cup cocoa powder
- ½ cup coconut oil
- 2 cups chopped pumpkin
- ½cup coconut flour
- ½ cup collagen protein powder
- 1 teaspoon baking soda
- 3teaspoons vanilla extract

Preparation:

1. Blend everything but the collagen.
2. When the pumpkin has blended completely, add the collagen and blitz again at the lowest possible speed.
3. Pour this mixture into the muffin tray and bake for 30 minutes.

Parmesan Cheese Crisps

Time: 10 minutes | Serves 6

Kcal: 32, Net carbs: 8% (0.3g / 0.01 oz) | Fiber: 1% (0.03g / 0.01 oz), Fat: 46% (2g / 0.07 oz) | Protein: 46% (2g / 0.07 oz)

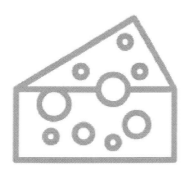

Ingredients:

♦ 1 cup shredded parmesan cheese
♦ 1 teaspoon basil (dried)

Preparation:

1. Prepare the baking sheet with a lining of parchment paper.
2. Place a spoonful of the shredded cheese on this paper and top it some dried basil. Repeat 11 times.
3. Bake for 6 minutes and serve!

Coffee Coconut Almond Smoothie

Time: 25 minutes | Serves 4

Kcal: 607, Net carbs: 6% (5g / 0.18 oz) | Fiber: 6% (5g / 0.18 oz), Fat: 53% (46g / 1.6 oz) | Protein: 35% (30g / 1.1 oz)

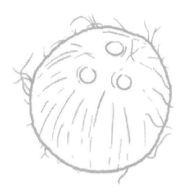

Ingredients:

♦ 6 ounces dark chocolate cold-brew coffee
♦ 2 scoops collagen protein powder
♦ 1 tablespoons of almond butter
♦ ¼ avocado
♦ ½ cupcoconut milk
♦ 1 teaspoon cocoa nibs
♦ 1 tablespoons of MCT oil
♦ ⅛ teaspoons sea salt
♦ ¼ teaspoons cinnamon

Preparation:

1. Blend all the ingredients except collagen protein for 30 seconds.
2. Add the collagen now at low speed and serve.

Peanut Butter Balls

Time: 20 minutes | Serves 18

Kcal: 193, Net carbs: 13% (4g / 0.14 oz) | Fiber: 10% (3g / 0.1 oz), Fat: 54% (17g / 0.6 oz) | Protein: 23% (7g / 0.3 oz)

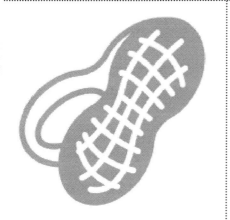

Ingredients:

- ♦ 8 ounces chocolate chips
- ♦ 1 cup peanut butter
- ♦ 1 cup chopped salted peanuts

Preparation:

1. Mix the peanut butter and peanuts to prepare the dough. Make 18 balls from it and put them on a baking sheet. Refrigerate.

2. Let the chocolate chips melt down.

3. Now dip the peanut butter balls in this dip and refrigerate again.

Raspberry Avocado Smoothie

Time: 4 minutes | Serves 2

Kcal: 223, Net carbs: 11% (4g / 0.14 oz) | Fiber: 25% (9g / 0.3 oz), Fat: 55% (20g / 0.7 oz) | Protein: 8% (3g / 0.1 oz)

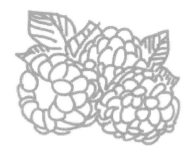

Ingredients:

- ♦ 1 pitted ripe avocado
- ♦ 2 tablespoons of lemon juice
- ♦ ½ cup frozen raspberries
- ♦ 1⅓ cup water
- ♦ 2 tablespoons of sweetener

Preparation:

1. Blend everything together and enjoy the freshness!

4 Weeks Diet Plan

If you are at loss about how to begin or where to start the keto diet, we are here to help! Let us walk you through the four-week-long diet plan with a new delicious recipe every day!

DAY 1

Breakfast:

Cream Cheese Pancakes

Serves 4 | 12 min

Kcal: 340, Net carbs: 6% (3g / 0.1 oz) | Fiber: 1% (1g / 0.03 oz) , Fat: 58% (30g / 1.1 oz) | Protein: 33% (17g / 0.6 oz)

Ingredients:

♦ 2 eggs

♦ 2 ounces cream cheese

♦ ½ teaspoons cinnamon

♦ 1 teaspoon sugar

♦ Berries

♦ Maple syrup

Preparation:

1. Blend everything till the mixture is consistent. Let it sit for a couple of minutes.

2. Spread this batter on a greased pan in portions of a quarter. Cook and flip till each side becomes golden.

3. Serve with maple syrup and berries.

Lunch: **Bacon and Olive Quiche** (Page-30)

Dinner: **Caprese Chicken** (Page-42)

DAY 2

Breakfast: **English Muffins** *(Page-18)*

Lunch:

Chicken Cucumber Avocado Salad

Serves 6 | 10 min

Kcal: 544, Net carbs: 6% (5g / 0.18 oz) | Fiber: 6% (5g / 0.18 oz), Fat: 43% (38g / 1.34 oz) | Protein: 45% (40g / 1.4 oz)

Ingredients:

- 1 deboned and shredded Rotisserie chicken
- ¼ thinly sliced onion
- 3 tablespoons of olive oil
- 4 chopped Roma tomatoes
- 2 diced avocados
- 1 sliced cucumber
- 3 tablespoons of lemon juice
- ½ cup chopped parsley
- Salt and pepper

Preparation:

1. Combine all the vegetables with chicken and parsley.
2. Toss it with salt and pepper, lemon juice and olive oil.
3. Serve fresh!

Dinner: **Shrimp and Sausage Skillet** *(Page-43)*

DAY 3

Breakfast: **Biscuits and Gravy** *(Page-19)*

Lunch: **Salmon and Avocado Salad** *(Page-31)*

Dinner:

Salsa Chicken Pot

Serves 6 | 35 min

Kcal: 243, Net carbs: 5% (3g / 0.1 oz) | Fiber: 4% (2g / 0.07 oz), Fat: 23% (10g / 0.35 oz) | Protein: 68% (30g / 1.1 oz)

Ingredients:

- 3 tablespoons of taco seasoning
- 4 ounces diced cream cheese
- 2 lbs. boneless chicken thighs
- ¼ cup chicken broth
- 1 cup salsa
- Salt and pepper

Preparation:

1. Arrange the chicken thighs at the bottom of your instant pot. Add the taco seasoning, cream cheese, broth, salsa, salt and pepper to it. Cook for about 20 minutes at a high temperature.

2. Let the pot release its pressure for about fifteen minutes.

3. Shred the chicken and put it in a bowl. Transfer the sauce into a blender and make a puree out of it. Coat the shredded chicken with this sauce.

DAY 4

Breakfast:

Eggs Benedict and Mug Bread

Serves 2 | 30min

Kcal: 600, Net carbs: 4% (3g / 0.1 oz) | Fiber: 3% (2g / 0.07 oz), Fat: 75% (60g / 2.12 oz) | Protein: 19% (15g / 0.5 oz)

Ingredients:

- 1 ounce smoked deli ham
- 3⅓ ounces butter
- 3 eggs
- 2 egg yolks
- 1 tablespoon of heavy whipping cream
- 1tablespoons of almond flour
- 1 tablespoon of coconut flour
- 1 tablespoon of lemon juice
- ¾ teaspoons baking powder
- Pepper
- 1 tablespoon of water
- 1 tablespoon of white vinegar
- 1 teaspoon salt

Preparation:

1. Take a glass bowl or cup with a flat bottom. Smear it with 1 teaspoon of butter to prepare the mug bread. Combine coconut flour, almond flower, an egg, baking powder, a teaspoon of whipped cream and a pinch of salt in this bowl. Stir the cream and mix it all again to prepare a smooth batter.

2. Bake it until the central part of bread is done.

3. When the mug bread cools down, take it out from the cup and cut in half.

4. To prepare the hollandaise sauce, let the butter first melt in the oven and then cool down.

5. Combine water and the egg yolks in a bowl. Now keep it inside a water bath and simmer. Stir repeatedly to have a thick consistency of sauce.

6. Take the pot out of the water bath. Slowly stir eggs after adding the melted butter and keep whisking.

7. Add lemon, pepper and salt for seasoning.

8. Mix a little bit of vinegar in a lot of water. Transfer it to a saucepan and let it simmer.

9. Crack open two eggs into the water one by one. Boil them in a low heat for a while.

10. Use a spoon to pick up the eggs and then place in cold water.Place them on a plate.

11. Fry the halved mug bread pieces with butter. Then place smoked ham, the cooked egg and the hollandaise sauce on each half. Serve fresh.

Lunch: **Cauliflower Potato Salad** *(Page-32)*

Dinner: **Spaghetti Squash Casserole** *(Page-44)*

DAY 5

Breakfast: **Goat Cheese Omelet with Vegetables** *(Page-20)*

Lunch:

Brussels Sprouts Salad with Vinaigrette

Serves 4 | 15 min

Kcal: 156, Net carbs: 24% (6g / 0.2 oz)| Fiber: 12% (3g / 0.1 oz), Fat: 54% (14g / 0.5 oz) | Protein: 12% (3g / 0.1 oz)

Ingredients:

♦ 1 lb. shaved brussels sprouts

♦ 4 sprigs thyme

♦ ¼ teaspoons whole grain mustard

♦ ½ lemon juiced

♦ ¼ cup olive oil

♦ ¼ teaspoons Dijon mustard

♦ 1 tablespoon of apple cider vinegar

♦ Sea salt

Preparation:

1. Simmer the sprouts 10 minutes in boiling water.

2. Prepare the vinaigrette by mixing all other ingredients except sea salt.

3. Drain the cooked sprouts and cool them down.

4. Toss them with vinaigrette and add sea salt for seasoning.

Dinner: **Mongolian Beef** *(Page-45)*

DAY 6

Breakfast: **French Pancakes** *(Page-21)*

Lunch: **Turkey with Cream Cheese Sauce** *(Page-33)*

Dinner:

Stuffed Salmon Rolls

Serves 4 | 30 min

Kcal: 399, Net carbs: 11% (8g / 0.3 oz)| Fiber: 1% (1g / 0.03 oz), Fat: 29% (22g / 0.78 oz) | Protein: 59% (44g / 1.55 oz)

Ingredients:

- ½ lb. trimmed asparagus
- 5 ounces salmon fillets
- ½ cup grated parmesan
- 2 tablespoons of chopped basil
- ½ cup chicken broth

- 2 tablespoons of lemon juice
- 2 teaspoons cornstarch
- 1 tablespoon of butter
- 2 teaspoons lemon zest
- Salt and pepper

Preparation:

1. Apply salt and pepper on salmon fillets for seasoning.

2. Mix parmesan, ricotta, lemon zest, basil, salt and pepper. Use this and the asparagus spears respectively as topping for the fillets.

3. Roll them up and bake at 425 Fahrenheit for 17 minutes.

4. Take a saucepan and melt the butter at medium heat. Combine broth, lemon juice and corn starch. Add this mixture with butter and cook for 4 minutes.

5. Top the salmon rolls with this lemon sauce and serve.

DAY 7

Breakfast:

Jalapeno Pepper Frittata

Serves 6 | 40 min

Kcal: 390, Net carbs: 12% (7g / 0.3 oz) | Fiber: 5% (3g / 0.1 oz), Fat: 54% (32g / 1.2 oz) | Protein: 29% (17g / 0.6 oz)

Ingredients:

♦ 7 eggs (large)
♦ 6 ounces chopped bacon
♦ 4 ounces cream cheese
♦ 3 jalapenos
♦ 2 minced garlic cloves
♦ 1 chopped medium cucumber
♦ 1 red bell pepper
♦ ¾ teaspoons salt
♦ 1 chopped Romaine lettuce head
♦ ½ teaspoons ground black pepper
♦ ¾ cup shredded cheddar cheese
♦ ⅓ cup heavy whipping cream

Preparation:

1. Cut one jalapeno into thin slices. Chop the other two jalapenos.

2. Sauté the bacon till they are crisp. Then spread them on a greased pie pan.

3. Sauté the garlic and chopped jalapenos for two minutes. Place these and cream cheese cubes on the pie pan over bacon.

4. Mix pepper, salt, cream and the eggs in a bowl. Pour this mixture on the pan and add cheddar cheese over the mixture. Bake for a few minutes.

5. Add the sliced jalapeno and bake again for 20 minutes.

6. Serve with cucumber, pepper and lettuce.

Lunch: **Fish Cakes with Avocado Lemon Dip** *(Page-34)*

Dinner: **Chicken Quesadillas** *(Page-47)*

DAY 8

Breakfast: Upma *(Page-22)*

Lunch:

Cauliflower Soup

Serves 6 | 40 min

Kcal: 469, Net carbs: 8% (6g / 0.2 oz) | Fiber: 5% (4g / 0.14 oz), Fat: 44% (34g / 1.66 oz) | Protein: 43% (33g / 1.64 oz)

Ingredients:

- 1 pack extra firm tofu, diced
- 6-8 pieces of cauliflower head (large)
- 1 quartered ginger
- 1 tablespoon of soy sauce
- ½ quartered carrot
- 8cups water
- 2 tablespoons of turmeric
- 2 cups coconut milk
- 2 teaspoons salt
- 1 tablespoon of olive oil
- 1 teaspoon smoked paprika
- Ground black pepper
- 1 teaspoon black pepper
- 1 teaspoon lemon juice
- ½ teaspoons of cumin

Preparation:

1. Sauté the carrots, cauliflower and ginger in boiling water for 20 minutes.

2. In another bowl, season the tofu cubes with cumin, olive oil, paprika, soy sauce and lemon juice. Bake them till they are brown and crisp.

3. When the vegetable soup cools down, blend it to get a smooth texture.

4. Cook this blended soup again with salt, pepper, turmeric and coconut milk.

Dinner: **Garlic Butter Salmon** *(Page-46)*

DAY 9

Breakfast: **Pumpkin Spice Latte** *(Page-23)*

Lunch: **Tuna Salad with Poached Eggs** *(Page-35)*

Dinner:

Sheet Pan Chicken and Vegetables

Serves 6 | 50 min

Kcal: 436, Net carbs: 7% (5g / 0.18 oz) | Fiber: 6% (4g / 0.14 oz), Fat: 43% (30g / 1.1 oz) | Protein: 43% (30g / 1.1 oz)

Ingredients:

- ♦ 2 minced garlic cloves
- ♦ ½ lb. quartered brussels sprouts
- ♦ 4 diced bacon slices
- ♦ 2 tablespoons of salted butter
- ♦ 6 chicken thighs
- ♦ ½ cups of cauliflower florets
- ♦ 2 tablespoons of avocado oil
- ♦ ½ teaspoons ground coriander
- ♦ ½ teaspoons paprika
- ♦ ⅛ teaspoons cayenne pepper
- ♦ 1 teaspoon black pepper
- ♦ ¾ teaspoons ground cumin
- ♦ 1½ teaspoons salt

Preparation:

1. Mix melted butter, cumin, coriander, paprika, cayenne, garlic, ½ teaspoons pepper and ¾ teaspoons salt. Use this mixture to brush over the chicken thighs.

2. In another bowl, combine sprouts, cauliflower, bacon and avocado oil with the rest of salt and pepper.

3. Arrange the vegetables on a baking sheet evenly. Top it with a layer of chicken thighs and bake for 37 minutes.

4. Broil the dish for 3 minutes until it turns brown.

DAY 10

Breakfast:

Soft Tortillas

Serves 12 | 35min

Kcal: 249, Net carbs: 5% (2g / 0.07 oz)| Fiber: 34% (15g / 0.5 oz), Fat: 48% (21g / 0.74 oz) | Protein: 14% (6g / 0.2 oz)

Ingredients:

♦ 6 large egg whites

♦ 2 cups coconut flour

♦ ½ teaspoons baking soda

♦ 3 cups hot water

♦ 1 cup olive oil

♦ 1 teaspoon salt

♦ ½ cup ground psyllium husk powder

Preparation:

1. Combine the flour, salt, psyllium husk and baking soda in a bowl.

2. Add olive oil and egg whites one by one. Make sure the mixture stays moist.

3. Add the hot water slowly with half-cup a time.

4. Make 12 balls out of this dough and flatten them like tortilla sheets.

5. Toast them in batches of two.

Lunch: **Cabbage Soup** *(Page-36)*

Dinner: **Chicken Quesadillas** *(Page-47)*

DAY 11

Breakfast: Scrambled Eggs with Veggies and Coconut Oil *(Page-24)*

Lunch:

Mediterranean Chicken Salad

Serves 4 | 25 min

Kcal: 335, Net carbs: 12% (7g / 0.3 oz) | Fiber: 10% (6g / 0.2 oz), Fat: 36% (21g / 0.74 oz) | Protein: 41% (24g / 0.85 oz)

Ingredients:

♦ 2 diced tomatoes

♦ 1 lb. boneless chicken breasts

♦ ⅓ cup sliced black olives

♦ 1 diced cucumber

♦ 4 cups lettuce

♦ 1 sliced red onion

♦ 1 sliced avocado

♦ 2 tablespoons of olive oil

♦ 2 tablespoons of red wine vinegar

♦ 2 tablespoons of chopped parsley

♦ ¼ cup lemon juice

♦ 2 teaspoons minced garlic

♦ 1 teaspoon salt 1 teaspoon dried oregano

♦ 2 tablespoons of water

♦ 2 teaspoons dried basil

♦ Pepper

Preparation:

1. Mix the chicken breasts with olive oil, lemon juice, vinegar, oregano, salt, pepper, parsley, basil and garlic. Refrigerate half of it for later and place the other half in a shallow dish.

2. Marinate the chicken in this shallow dish with the mixture and let it sit for an hour.

3. In another bowl, combine lettuce, tomatoes, cucumber, avocado, onion and black olives.

4. Grill the marinated chicken in 1 tablespoon of oil at medium-high heat.

5. Cut the grilled chicken into slices before placing it on the salad. Serve with the refrigerated dressing.

Dinner: **Greek Shrimp** *(Page-48)*

DAY 12

Breakfast: **Cornbread** *(Page-25)*

Lunch: **Indian Chicken Lettuce Wrap** *(Page-37)*

Dinner:

Buttered Cod

Serves 4 | 10 min

Kcal: 293, Net carbs: 2% (1g / 0.03 oz) | Fiber: 2% (1g / 0.03 oz), Fat: 36% (18g / 0.6 oz) | Protein: 60% (30g / 1.1 oz)

Ingredients:

- 1½ lbs. cod fillets
- ¼ teaspoons ground pepper
- ¾ teaspoons ground paprika
- ½ teaspoons salt
- ¼ teaspoons garlic powder
- 6 tablespoons of sliced unsalted butter
- Lemon slices
- Parsley

Preparation:

1. Combine everything except the fish and butter to prepare the seasoning.
2. Use it to brush all sides of each fillet.
3. Melt 2 tablespoons of butter in a skillet and cook cod in it for a couple of minutes.
4. Lower the heat, cook for three minutes after adding the remaining butter.
5. When the butter melts down, transfer the cod in a plate. Top it with parsley and lemon juice before serving.

DAY 13

Breakfast:

Eggs with Tarragon Chive Cream Sauce

Serves 4 | 25min

Kcal: 400, Net carbs: 5% (3g / 0.1 oz)| Fiber: 0% (0g / 0 oz), Fat: 60% (35g / 1.23 oz) | Protein: 34% (20g / 0.7 oz)

Ingredients:

- ♦ 1 cup heavy whipping cream
- ♦ 8 eggs (large)
- ♦ 2pinches ground nutmeg
- ♦ 2minced garlic cloves
- ♦ 2 teaspoons chopped chives

- ♦ 2 teaspoons chopped tarragon
- ♦ ½ cup grated parmesan cheese
- ♦ ½ teaspoons ground black pepper
- ♦ ½ teaspoons sea salt

Preparation:

1. Place four oiled 8-ounce ramekins on the baking sheet.

2. Mix cream, tarragon, chives, cheese, garlic, nutmeg, salt and pepper to pre-pare the sauce. Put it into the ramekins.

3. Add two eggs to each ramekin as topping.

4. Bake for about 15 minutes.

Lunch: **Cheesy Taco Skillet** *(Page-38)*

Dinner: **Bacon Brie Frittata** *(Page-49)*

DAY 14

Breakfast: Overnight Coconut Chia Pudding *(Page-26)*

Lunch:

Cauliflower Grits with Arugula and Shrimp

Serves 4 | 30 min

Kcal: 305, Net carbs: 15% (8g / 0.3 oz) | Fiber: 9% (5g / 0.18 oz) | Fat: 33% (18g / 0.6 oz) | Protein: 44% (24g / 0.85 oz)

Ingredients:

- 1 cup whole milk
- 1 lb. deveined shrimp
- 1 tablespoon of extra-virgin olive oil
- 4 cups riced cauliflower
- 3sliced garlic cloves
- 1 tablespoon of unsalted butter
- 1 tablespoon of paprika
- ½ cup crumbled goat cheese
- 4 cups baby arugula
- Ground black pepper
- 2 teaspoons garlic powder
- ½ teaspoons cayenne pepper
- Salt

Preparation:

1. Combine cayenne, garlic powder and paprika. Coat this mixture over the shrimp and then refrigerate it.

2. Prepare the cauliflower rice with butter by cooking for 2 minutes.

3. Add half cup of milk and boil on low heat for 7 minutes.

4. Now add rest of the milk and simmer for 10 more minutes.

5. Add goat cheese, salt and pepper to finish off the cauliflower grits.

6. Sauté the garlic for a minute in olive oil. Introduce the arugula and continue for 4 minutes. Top it with pepper and salt before removing.

7. Sauté the shrimp in this same bowl for 5 minutes using olive oil. Add salt and pepper for seasoning.

8. Serve a quarter of each dish on a plate.

Dinner: **Asian Steak** *(Page-50)*

DAY 15

Breakfast: **Chai Latte** *(Page-27)*

Lunch: **Drumsticks with Chili Aioli** *(Page-39)*

Dinner:

Cheesy Bacon Spinach

Serves 6 | 30 min

Kcal: 327, Net carbs: 4% (2g / 0.07 oz) | Fiber: 2% (1g / 0.03 oz), Fat: 53% (27g / 0.95 oz) | Protein: 41% (21g / 0.74 oz)

Ingredients:

- 6 chopped bacon strips
- 5 ounces baby spinach
- 2 minced garlic cloves
- 6 boneless chicken thighs
- ½ cup crumbled feta
- 1 cup heavy cream
- 1 tablespoon of butter
- ½ cup grated Parmesan
- Salt and pepper

Preparation:

1. Cook the bacon till its crisp and then drain while reserving the grease in the pan.

2. Brush the thighs with salt and pepper. Cook them in the grease, each side for 4 minutes.

3. Melt the butter and cook garlic in it for a minute. Sauté spinach in this fragrant mixture for 2 minutes.

4. Add parmesan and heavy cream. Cook this for 3 minutes.

5. Return the bacon and chicken into this thick sauce. Stir thoroughly and spread some crumbled feta on it.

DAY 16

Breakfast

Dairy-Free Latte

Serves 4 | 5 min

Kcal: 190, Net carbs: 4% (1g / 0.03 oz) | Fiber: 0% (0g / 0 oz), Fat: 72% (18g / 0.6 oz) | Protein: 24% (6g / 0.2 oz)

Ingredients:

- ♦ 2 pinches vanilla extract
- ♦ 3 cups boiling water
- ♦ 4 tablespoons of coconut oil
- ♦ 4 eggs
- ♦ 2 teaspoons ground ginger

Preparation:

1. Blend everything together and drink fresh!

Lunch: **Bacon and Olive Quiche** *(Page-30)*

Dinner: **Caprese Chicken** *(Page-42)*

DAY 17

Breakfast: **English Muffins** *(Page-18)*

Lunch:

Sushi

Serves 2 | 20 min

Kcal: 230, Net carbs: 14% (5g / 0.18 oz) | Fiber: 11% (4g / 0.14 oz), Fat: 63% (22g / 0.78 oz) | Protein: 11% (4g / 0.14 oz)

Ingredients:

♦ 1.5 ounces cream cheese

♦ ½ sliced avocado

♦ 1 tablespoon of coconut oil

♦ 1 cup chopped cauliflower

♦ ¼ cup sliced cucumber

Preparation:

1. Blend a fifth of the cauliflower florets to use them as rice.

2. Cook it with coconut oil for 6 minutes. Transfer it to a bowl.

3. Spread the rice in on layer on a nori wrapper. Then layer it with avocado, cucumber and cheese.

4. Roll the wrap and cut it into 8 sushi pieces. Start cutting from the middle for convenience.

Dinner: **Shrimp and Sausage Skillet** *(Page-43)*

DAY 18

Breakfast: **Goat Cheese Omelet with Vegetables** *(Page-20)*

Lunch: **Salmon and Avocado Salad** *(Page-31)*

Dinner:

Sesame Tofu and Eggplant

Serves 4 | 15 min

Kcal: 293, Net carbs: 15% (7g / 0.3 oz) | Fiber: 11% (5g / 0.18 oz), Fat: 51% (24g / 0.85 oz) | Protein: 23% (11g / 0.4 oz)

Ingredients:

- 1 teaspoons crushed red pepper flakes
- 1 lb sliced tofu
- ¼ cup soy sauce
- 3 tablespoons of rice vinegar
- Salt and pepper
- 1 julienned eggplant
- 2 minced garlic cloves
- 1 cup chopped cilantro
- ¼ cup sesame seeds
- 2 teaspoons sweetener
- 4 tablespoons of toasted sesame oil
- 1 tablespoon of olive oil

Preparation:

1. Mix minced garlic, red pepper flakes, sweetener, a quarter of the cilantro and half the toasted sesame oil together. Use this to marinate the eggplant.

2. Cook the marinated eggplant in olive oil.

3. Stir in the rest of cilantro and transfer it to the serving plate.

4. Coat the tofu slices with sesame seeds. Fry them in 2 tablespoons of sesame oil until they turn crisp.

5. Add ¼ cup soy sauce to coat the tofu. Cook till they become brown.

6. Serve the eggplants with these tofu on top.

DAY 19

Breakfast

Naan with garlic butter

Serves 8 | 25 min

Kcal: 219, Net carbs: 3% (1g / 0.03 oz) | Fiber: 22% (7g / 0.3 oz), Fat: 68% (22g / 0.78 oz) | Protein: 6% (2g / 0.07 oz)

Ingredients:

- ½ teaspoons baking powder
- ¾ cup coconut flour
- 4 ounces butter
- 2 tablespoons of ground psyllium husk powder 2 cups boiling water
- ⅓ cup melted coconut oil
- 2minced garlic cloves
- 1 teaspoon salt
- Sea salt

Preparation:

1. Mix all the dry ingredients with oil and some boiling water. Stir thoroughly to get a smooth texture.
2. Break up the dough into 8 portions and flatten to serve as naan.
3. Fry each piece until it gets a beautiful golden hue.
4. Heat up the butter to melt. Add the minced garlic and stir.
5. Apply the garlic butter sauce on each naan with a brush. You can add some salt on top.
6. Serve the naan pieces using rest of the garlic butter as a dip.

Lunch: **Cauliflower Potato Salad** *(Page-32)*

Dinner: **Spaghetti Squash Casserole** *(Page-44)*

DAY 20

Breakfast: Upma *(Page-22)*

Lunch:

Lemon Balsamic Chicken

Serves 6 | 35 min

Kcal: 322, Net carbs: 5% (3g / 0.1 oz) | Fiber: 7% (4g / 0.14 oz), Fat: 33% (18g / 0.6 oz) | Protein: 54% (29g / 1 oz)

Ingredients:

- 2 lbs boneless chicken thighs
- 2 bay leaves
- 2 tablespoons of lemon rind (minced)
- 1 cup shredded purple cabbage
- 1 cup sliced onion
- 5 tablespoons of olive oil

- 3 tablespoons of pastured butter
- 1½ tablespoons of balsamic vinegar
- 2 teaspoons salt
- 1 teaspoon coarse black pepper
- 1 teaspoon dried herb

Preparation:

1. Sauté the onion, cabbage and lemon in 2 tablespoons of butter.

2. Now add the chicken, bay leaves and seasoning ingredients. Cook this concoction for 3 minutes.

3. Add the vinegar and cook under pressure for 20 minutes.

4. Add the rest of the butter and stir.

Dinner: Mongolian Beef *(Page-45)*

DAY 21

Breakfast: **Cornbread** *(Page-25)*

Lunch: **Turkey with Cream Cheese Sauce** *(Page-33)*

Dinner:

Pizza Chicken

Serves 6 | 35 min

Kcal: 440, Net carbs: 4% (3g / 0.1 oz) | Fiber: 1% (1g / 0.03 oz), Fat: 40% (27g / 0.95 oz) | Protein: 53% (36g / 1.27 oz)

Ingredients:

♦ 2 lbs boneless chicken thighs

♦ 2 cups mozzarella (shredded)

♦ 2 ounces sliced pepperoni

♦ 1 cup marinara sauce

♦ 2 tablespoons of olive oil

♦ Salt and pepper

Preparation:

1. Sprinkle pepper and salt on the chicken for seasoning. Cook each side of it for 3 minutes using olive oil on a skillet. Add the pizza sauce to coat.

2. Top the chicken with layers of pepperoni and chicken. Bake them for about 30 minutes and put it in the broiler for 2 minutes.

DAY 22

Breakfast:

Garlic Rosemary Focaccia

Serves 4 | 35 min

Kcal: 205, Net carbs: 7% (2g / 0.07 oz)| Fiber: 0% (0g / 0 oz), Fat: 66% (19g / 0.7 oz) | Protein: 28% (8g / 0.3 oz)

Ingredients:

- 1 egg
- 1½ cups shredded mozzarella cheese
- 2 tablespoons of cream cheese
- 2 ounces butter
- 3 chopped garlic cloves
- 1 teaspoon white wine vinegar
- ¾ cup almond flour
- ½ teaspoons chopped rosemary
- ½ teaspoons salt
- ½ teaspoons sea salt
- ½ teaspoons garlic powder

Preparation:

1. Melt cream and mozzarella cheese in an oven or a pan. Don't let it stick.

2. Stir in vinegar, egg, almond flour, garlic powder and salt to prepare the dough.

3. Flatten the dough a little to resemble focaccia structure. Place them on parchment paper.

4. Use a fork to make holes in it and bake until it turns golden.

5. In a separate bowl combine garlic, rosemary, salt and butter. After the bread is baked, spread this mixture on top.

6. Put it back in the oven for another 10 minutes.

Lunch: **Fish Cakes with Avocado Lemon Dip** *(Page-34)*

Dinner: **Loaded Cauliflower** *(Page-51)*

DAY 23

Breakfast: Coffee Coconut Almond Smoothie *(Page-56)*

Lunch:

White Beef Chili

Serves 5 | 15 minutes

Kcal: 385, Net carbs: 9% (6g / 0.2 oz) | Fiber: 3% (2g / 0.07 oz), Fat: 47% (30g / 1.1 oz) | Protein: 45% (29g / 1 oz)

Ingredients:

- 2 garlic cloves (minced)
- 2 tablespoons of coconut oil
- 2 cups riced cauliflower
- Salt and black pepper
- 2 cups heavy cream
- ½ onion (minced)

- 1 tablespoons of mustard
- 1teaspoons thyme
- 1 teaspoon celery
- 1 lb. ground beef
- 1 teaspoon garlic powder

Preparation:

1. Cook the minced onion and garlic in coconut oil for 3 minutes.

2. Add the beef, break it down and stir thoroughly.

3. Add the previously prepared seasoning mix and the riced cauliflower.

4. When the beef turns brown, add coconut milk. When it starts to simmer, stir for 8 minutes in low heat.

Dinner: **Spaghetti Squash Casserole** *(Page-44)*

DAY 24

Breakfast: **Overnight Coconut Chia Pudding** *(Page-26)*
Lunch: **Tuna Salad with Poached Eggs** *(Page-35)*
Dinner:

Beef Bourguignon

Serves 6 | 50 min

Kcal: 265, Net carbs: 6% (3g / 0.1 oz)| Fiber: 13% (7g / 0.3 oz), Fat: 35% (18g / 0.6 oz) | Protein: 46% (24g / 0.85 oz)

Ingredients:

- 2 lbs diced beef chuck roast
- 10 ounces quartered cremini mushrooms
- 5 diced bacon strips
- 1 teaspoon thyme (dried)
- 5 garlic cloves (minced)
- 1 chopped onion
- 2 chopped carrots
- 3 bay leaves
- 1 tablespoon of tomato paste
- ¾ cup dry red wine
- ¾ teaspoons xanthan gum
- Salt and pepper

Preparation:

1. Season with pepper and salt (the beef). Now sauté them with a pressure cooker and then set aside.

2. Add diced bacon to the same container and cook for 5 minutes more. Put it on a plate.

3. Cook the beef in a pot until it turns brown. Put it on a plate.

4. Add garlic and onions. Keep cooking.

5. Add the red wine and the tomato paste. Stir thoroughly and make sure the tomato paste has dissolved.

6. Return the beef to pot. Add mushrooms, bay leaves, thyme and the carrots. Cook for 40 minutes at high pressure with the lid on.

7. Take the bay leaves out and add xanthan gum to the dish. Stew for a minute.

8. Serve with crispy bacon.

DAY 25

Breakfast

Cornbread Waffles with Bacon and Egg

Serves 8 | 15 min

Kcal: 323, Net carbs: 2% (1g / 0.03 oz) | Fiber: 10% (5g / 0.18 oz), Fat: 65% (31g / 1.2 oz) | Protein: 23% (11g / 0.4 oz)

Ingredients:

- 4 ounces melted butter
- 4 ounces chopped cooked bacon
- 4 eggs
- ⅓ cup oat fibre
- ¼ cup coconut flour
- 1½ teaspoons baking powder
- ¼ cup water
- ⅓ cup melted coconut oil
- ½ cup cheddar cheese
- ⅓ cup unflavored whey protein isolate
- 2 chopped scallions

Preparation:

1. Combine all the dry components first. Then start adding the water, butter, coconut oil and the eggs and stir.

2. Beat the mixture. Add cheese, bacon and scallions.

3. Use this as the waffle dough and place accordingly into a waffle iron. Remember not to go overboard with the portions.

4. When the waffles turn brown, serve warm and fresh!

Lunch: **Cabbage Soup** *(Page-36)*

Dinner: **Asian Steak** *(Page-50)*

DAY 26

Breakfast: **Raspberry Avocado Smoothie** *(Page-58)*

Lunch:

Avocado and Shrimp Wrap

Serves 2 | 20 min

Kcal: 1003, Net carbs: 7% (10g / 0.35 oz) | Fiber: 10% (15g / 0.5 oz), Fat: 63% (91g / 3.2 oz) | Protein: 19% (28g / 1 oz)

Ingredients:

- 1 ounce butter
- 6 ounces cooked shrimp
- 4 eggs
- ¼ cup parsley
- 2 diced avocados
- 1 sliced celery stalk

- ½ cup mayonnaise
- ½ diced apple
- 1 teaspoon lemon juice
- 1 teaspoons chilli paste
- Salt and pepper

Preparation:

1. Whisk the eggs with pepper and salt. Cook half of it on melted butter. When the wrap is firm enough, transfer it to a plate. Repeat the process with the rest of the butter.

2. Toss the diced avocado with lime juice. Combine it with apple, celery, mayonnaise, parsley and chilli paste.

3. Coat the cooked shrimp with this mixture. Use pepper and salt for it to taste better.

Dinner: **Loaded Cauliflower** *(Page-51)*

DAY 27

Breakfast: **French Pancakes** *(Page-21)*

Lunch: **Salmon and Avocado Salad** *(Page-31)*

Dinner:

Chicken Enchilada Soup

Serves 8 | 40 min

Kcal: 311, Net carbs: 10% (5g / 0.18 oz) | Fiber: 2% (1g / 0.03 oz), Fat: 31% (16g / 0.6 oz) | Protein: 57% (29g / 1 oz)

Ingredients:

♦ 2 lbs boneless chicken breasts

♦ 5 cups chicken breasts

♦ ¾ cup sour cream

♦ 2 cups pureed tomatoes

♦ 2 diced jalapenos

♦ ¼ cup butter

♦ ½ cup chopped onion

♦ ¾ teaspoons salt

♦ 3 tablespoons of taco seasoning

Preparation:

1. Take a slow cooker or an instant pot. Add chicken, jalapenos, tomatoes, onion, broth, taco seasoning, butter and salt. Cook as soup for 20 minutes (for instant pot) or 7 hours (for slow cooker).

2. Put the chicken on a separate plate. Now take 1 cup of its broth in a bowl. Add sour cream to it and whisk well. Pour the creamy mixture in the pot.

3. Shred the chicken and return this to the pot as well.

4. Serve the delicious meal with cheese.

DAY 28

Breakfast

Soft Seed Bread

Serves 10 | 50 min

Kcal: 222, Net carbs: 6% (2g / 0.07 oz) | Fiber: 15% (5g / 0.18 oz), Fat: 60% (20g / 0.7 oz) | Protein: 18% (6g / 0.2 oz)

Ingredients:

- 3½ ounces cream cheese (room temperature)
- 3 eggs
- ½ teaspoons ground caraway seeds
- 1½ teaspoons baking powder
- ½ cup almond flour
- ¼ cup melted coconut oil
- 6 tablespoons of coconut flour
- 6tablespoons of heavy whipping cream
- 2 tablespoons of ground psyllium husk powder
- 4 tablespoons of sesame seeds
- ½ teaspoons salt

Preparation:

1. Combine every dry ingredient except for the seeds.

2. In another bowl, whisk the other ingredients for a smooth batter.

3. Now add the dry mixture to it.

4. Bake this dough for 45 minutes.

Lunch: **Indian Chicken Lettuce Wraps** *(Page-37)*

Dinner: **Shrimp and Sausage Skillet** *(Page-43)*

EXCLUSIVE BONUS!

Get Keto Audiobook for FREE NOW!*

The Ultimate Keto Diet Guide 2019-2020:
How to Loose weight with Quick and Easy Steps

SCAN ME

or go to

www.free-keto.co.uk

Disclaimer

The opinions and ideas of the author contained in this publication are designed to educate the reader in an informative and helpful manner. While we accept that the instructions will not suit every reader, it is only to be expected that the recipes might not gel with everyone. Use the book responsibly and at your own risk. This work with all its contents, does not guarantee correctness, completion, quality or correctness of the provided information. Always check with your medical practitioner should you be unsure whether to follow a low carb eating plan. Misinformation or misprints cannot be completely eliminated. Human error is real!

Coverphoto: Larisa Blinova

Printed in Great Britain
by Amazon